Bringing Back Yvette

John Gurley

AuthorHouse™
1663 Liberty Drive
Bloomington, IN 47403
www.authorhouse.com
Phone: 1 (800) 839-8640

Published by AuthorHouse 02/06/2015

ISBN: 978-1-4969-6847-0 (sc)
ISBN: 978-1-4969-6868-5 (e)

Library of Congress Control Number: 2015901968

Any people depicted in stock imagery provided by Thinkstock are models,
and such images are being used for illustrative purposes only.
Certain stock imagery © Thinkstock.

This book is printed on acid-free paper.

authorHOUSE®

Introduction

This is my fourth book about my wife, Yvette, who was in a Memory Support unit of a Care Center that is part of Vi at Palo Alto, a large luxury retirement home. The three previous books, starting with Vignettes of Yvette at Vi, were also published by Authorhouse. Those three books were written when Yvette was still alive. This fourth one, unfortunately, was written after her death. The title of this one has two meanings. First, Carmen (Yvette's wonderful caregiver) and I did bring her back from the almost-dead, which was initially explained in the third book, Even More Vignettes of Yvette at Vi. We continue that story here. (Can you now guess the title of the second book?) Second, we wish to bring Yvette back with memories of her during her last several months of life in Memory Support. We brought her back once, physically. Now we shall try to bring her back using our memories.

1

"We all know it was not the ugly Dementia Beast that devoured Yvette. No. It was the beautiful Sleep Fairy who decided to close our Darling's eyelids forever and ever."

That is what we wish to believe. But it is not true. That hideous Beast got her. The Sleep Fairy was shunted to the side.

2

Yvette fought the Dementia Beast courageously each time it struck. The Beast took away the use of her legs, but Yvette adapted beautifully, without complaint, to a transport chair. She sat in it like a Queen. The Beast began curling her fingers and soon rendered her hands all but useless. Once more, Yvette learned quickly how to hold the "burritos" Carmen made for her, how to hold out her fist in a threatening or a friendly way, and how to enjoy her food while being fed by Carmen. This damnable Dementia Beast next removed most of her ability to speak. Yvette overcame much of this by learning how to communicate with Carmen and me in several other ways. She used her eyes most effectively. However, when the Beast continually poured mucus into her throat and esophagus and removed some instructions on how to swallow it, Yvette was left with no effective response. Of course, she fought this one, too, for nearly to the end she willed to live. But the Beast had finally found the way to kill her. Yvette's heart eventually just stopped from the impossible demands on it. Our Beauty Queen was no more.

3

On Tuesday morning, December 9, 2014, at 9:25, I left Carmen alone with Yvette to go to the bathroom. During my 5 minute absence, Carmen saw Yvette open her eyes for the first time that morning, and she looked very strange. Carmen, startled, yelled for the nurse to come in fast. I returned at 9:30 as the nurse announced that Yvette was dead. I rushed to her bedside, and then Yvette breathed in deeply, let her breath out, and then she died. I saw and heard Yvette take her last breath. Carmen told me later that Yvette waited until I had returned before dying.

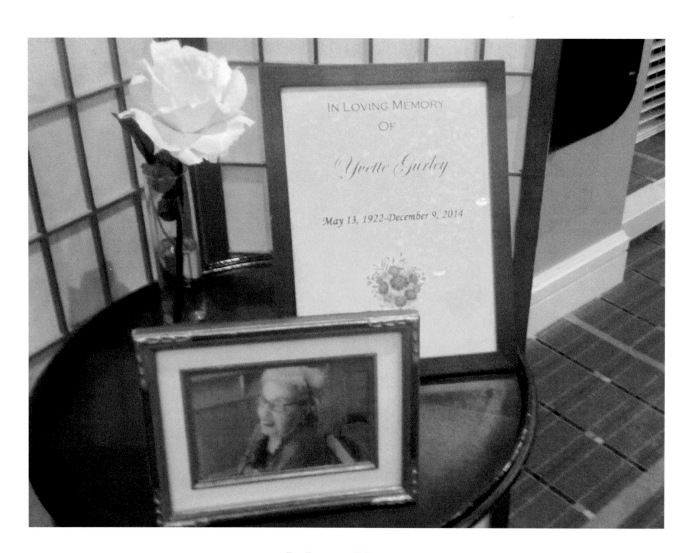

In Loving Memory

4

The day before Yvette died, she knew she was dying. I had held her hand during every day but two since she had been in Memory Support, and that's 975 times. While holding hands, we have at times smiled at each other, mostly we were simply relaxed and were content with the simple thing we were doing, and occasionally my story-telling was designed to elicit some hand response from her. However, the day before Yvette died, I sat next to her, reached under the covers, and found her hand. In a minute, Yvette began to cry, something I had not ever seen before. Tears came out of both corners of her eyes. Carmen came over with a damp cloth and began wiping away the tear drops. But there were more, as Yvette continued the weeping. At this point in her life, Yvette was not able to say much. She could not tell me, in the ordinary way, that we were about to part and that she was saddened by it. So she did what she could: she cried as we held hands. When I remembered this the next morning, just after my dear wife had passed on, I reached out, held her hand, and then it was I who cried.

5

Three days before Yvette died, she had her last meal with Carmen, a Saturday night dinner. Carmen told me the next day that, during the entire dinner, Yvette never took her eyes off of her. With her eyes, Yvette followed Carmen when she got up to prepare the next dish, looked into Carmen's eyes as she was being fed. Finally, Carmen, nearly unnerved, asked Yvette if there was something she wanted to tell her. Carmen had tears in her eyes as Yvette just continued to look at her. After she died a few days later, Carmen and I wondered if Yvette knew then that she would soon lose her very best friend.

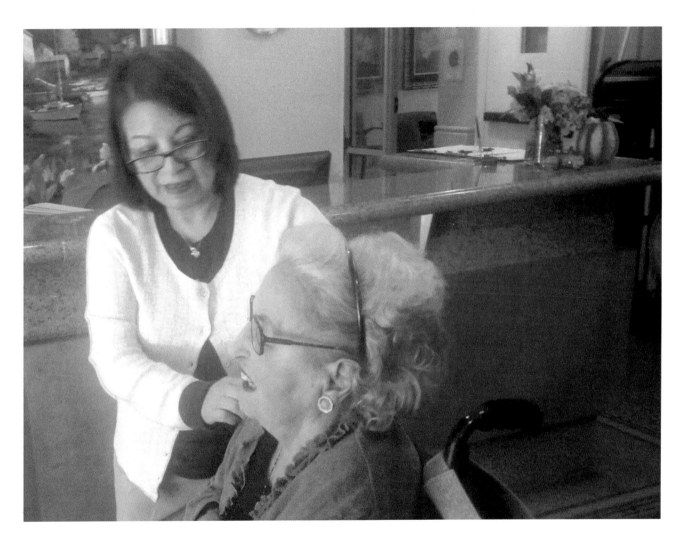

Carmen and Yvette

6

How did Yvette know she was dying? Simple. Carmen, I, her doctor, and a nurse or two, discussed at various times in Yvette's presence her deteriorating condition. In doing that, we made a huge mistake. We never should have done that. Carmen and I knew that Yvette was often listening to our talk and that she could understand the meaning of the conversation. She simply wasn't able to respond to it in any ordinary way. But she heard and she knew. She did respond by the only means left to her, with her eyes and with tears. She used her eyes to tell Carmen goodbye. She used her tears to tell me goodbye.

7

I took a picture of Yvette a few minutes after she died. As you can see, she died serenely, peacefully, without stress, colorfully, in her own bed, next to Andy Warhol's flowers, with a "burrito" in her right hand, held straight up. For some reason, which I find impossible to explain, it's the burrito that keeps haunting me day and night. Even while dying, Yvette followed Carmen's daily instruction to keep holding it. Maybe she was showing that to us by holding it straight up.

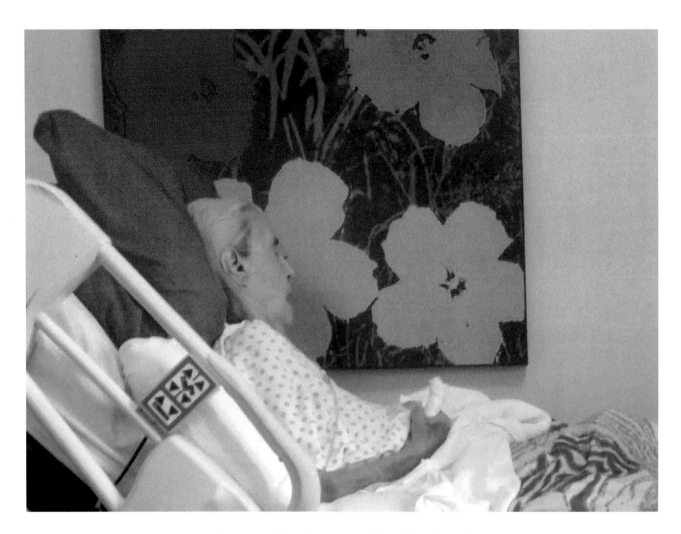

Yvette, a Few Minutes After Her Death

8

After Yvette died, I received many cards and notes in which the writer expressed condolences at Yvette's passing. Not one of them -- not one -- noted that Yvette died. "Passing" indicates that she is going somewhere, that nothing is yet final, the event is still going on. Most of the sympathizers probably meant that Yvette was passing from the Earth to Heaven -- and that it takes a little time.

One young woman, the day after Yvette died, told me that Yvette was now looking down at me and laughing at my grieving for her, for she was happier than she had ever been.

Why would I be in grief?, this young woman wanted to know. Well, I might ask, how come, on a globe, with everyone pointing up to a different part of the sky, each believes she knows where Heaven is? Well, maybe Heaven is everywhere. If so, how did Yvette get so quickly into a position to see me? If Heaven is everywhere, I could not be seen from most of Heaven.

Yvette died. If I have to grieve, it's because I miss her so very much. If she is happier than she has ever been, wonderful! But I am still completely lost without her. Let me grieve.

9

Among Yvette's many friends, there were a large number of just ordinary, but very fine, working people. Many of the sanitation workers at the Stanford Shopping Center, the servers and the hostess in the restaurant at Neiman Marcus, the clerks in La Baguette, the room cleaners, dishwasher, food deliverers, and others in Memory Support, nurse's aides in Assisted Living, workers in Skilled Nursing, and some cleaning women at Vi. All of them have expressed to Carmen and me their deep love for Yvette. When told of Yvette's death, the faces of all these workers showed great sorrow, and many cried. Our Beauty Queen, who often moved so regally among them, nevertheless captured their love with her magnificent smile, her beauty, and her politeness. I'm sure that some also admired her determination to know who they were, to learn their names.

10

My wife was more beautiful in the last four months of her life than she had ever been. I'm talking about the months right after her long recoveries from two pneumonias. Right then, after dropping 20 pounds during her struggles for survival. Right then, after missing the beauty salon for 14 weeks. Indeed, after fighting back, recapturing a few of those lost pounds, letting her hair turn whatever color it would, Yvette was then at the peak of her beauty, more strikingly pretty than she had been at 20, 40, or any earlier age.

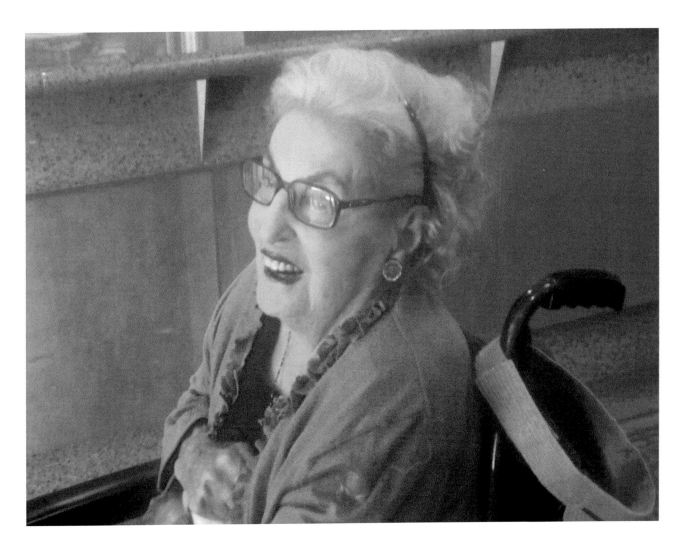

Our Beauty Queen

STOP. I really do not want to hear that beauty is in the eye of the beholder. STOP. Please keep your remarks about the blindness of a husband's love for his wife to yourselves. I'm telling you that by international beauty standards Yvette was a clear winner. At the age of 92. Did you get that? At 92! After a horrible battle to stay alive. After being bedridden for weeks. Out of all that emerged this Beauty Queen, with such a dazzling smile and gorgeous blonde golden hair and such a clear and healthy complexion, without a wrinkle on her face, and a miraculous X factor that we all knew was there, but could not explain. Permit me once more to declare that my wife, during the last four months of her life, was simply beautiful.

I know that this was so, but I do not know how or why. Where did that stunning golden blonde hair come from? Certainly not from artificial coloring. Not from her younger days, for Yvette grew up a brunette. Even so, suppose she had been a blonde at age 3, by what magic would the blonde hair have come back? Everyone who saw her during her last months commented on her lovely, bright, golden hair, which played such a large role in displaying her pretty looks. And those rosy cheeks? Not from applied rouge. They came to her out of her fight for survival. How did that happen? And those brilliant smiles? Of course, her smile was always her stock in trade, but how was she capable of producing so many of them, after so much was taken out of her during those two illnesses and recoveries? How come she was then at the peak of her beauty?

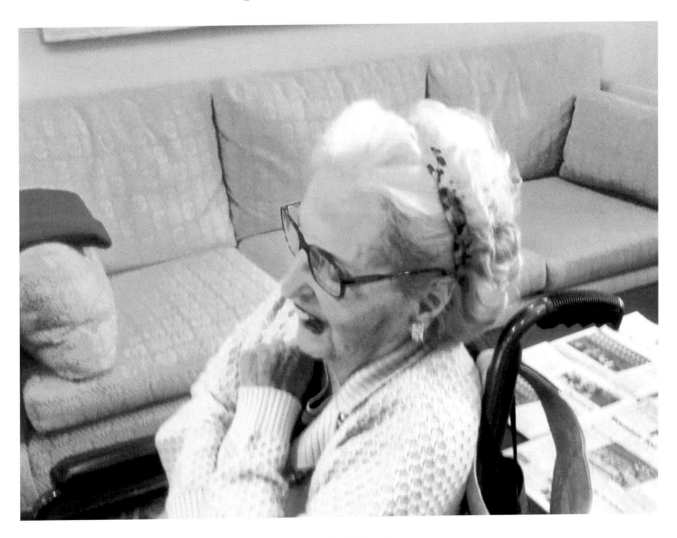

At the Peak of Her Beauty

In trying to explain it, Carmen and I may have taken flight from the sensible by supposing that an Angel came down from Heaven with her golden wand, with instructions to render our Darling more beautiful than she had ever been. This Angel, with one touch of her wand on Yvette's hair, a second touch on her cheeks, and then a gentle wave of the wand around Yvette's head, accomplished her mission, and flew back into the clouds. We even believe that Yvette herself willed this -- that she was so grateful to us for bringing her back to good health that she asked an Angel to make her more beautiful than ever for our own pleasure. How else could she meet this obligation? Really, something like that had to occur, for we have found no-one yet who can give us a better explanation of this miracle. Several have been offered, but none accords with what we know about Yvette. So we say Angel. Let's hear it, if you have something better.

11

During Yvette's long stay (977 days) in Memory Support, she had her hair done in the Care Center's Beauty Salon, by the beautician Carmen Ayon. After Yvette recovered from her two pneumonias, not having gone to the Salon for 14 weeks, her hair was golden blonde and truly beautiful. I emphasize again that that's the way it just naturally grew out during her recovery periods. Carmen Galindo began to take Yvette back to the Salon on Monday mornings for a hair wash, perhaps a haircut, and curling and waving. No coloring. On one of these Monday mornings, Carmen Ayon was beginning to curl and wave Yvette's hair, when two other women who had finished and were about to depart, suddenly announced that they simply had to stay to see Yvette's gorgeous hair once Carmen had finished. So there they sat for the next 15 minutes, admiring the growing beauty of Yvette's golden hair, as Carmen finished the job. Then they left with many words of admiration for what they had seen. Our beautician later told us that that had never happened to her before.

12

In the Memory Support units, the nursing staff comprises about 30 people originally from all over the world, men and women, some with accents of various kinds, many different skin colors on display, various ways of doing a job. Every day Carmen needed help to get Yvette in or out of bed, into the bathroom, changing her diapers, getting meals set up, and so on. So each day Yvette saw Carmen with several people, who might be different from the day before, and who could be different tomorrow. Yvette handled this problem by always looking intently at the name tags of the people helping her. While someone was helping Carmen lift Yvette into her chair, Yvette's head was turned to where his or her name tag should be. All of these workers learned to accommodate Yvette's curiosity by displaying their tags in easily observable places, or, in the case of some women, keeping their hair from hiding their tags, or helping Yvette by telling her who's who, or even giving hints. Knowing Yvette's penchant for wanting to know who this guy is, some of the workers challenged Yvette, even when she was just being wheeled around, to read their name tags. Yvette always took a look but seldom responded -- seldom was able to respond. We all remember, though, when Yvette, so challenged, came out with "Francesca" and, later, "Ernesto." Whether Yvette responded or not, she seems to have had this crew pretty well sorted out.

13

Roberta (not her real name) is in her 90s and was in Memory Support 2 along with my wife, Yvette, 8 other women, and 2 men. Roberta loved to wander around and often strayed into rooms not her own, sometimes just looking around. But she would also take what she could, use the bathroom, or settle down on the sofa. Carmen, who cared for Yvette for 2 1/2 years, often chased her out of Yvette's room and bathroom.

Yvette required, a few times each day, a breathing treatment that involved wearing a nose-and-mouth mask with a liquid in a container attached to the mask. The liquid was turned into a vapor by a machine hooked to the mask by a long rubber tube. When the treatment was running its course, the machine was making a racket and Yvette, who felt uncomfortable wearing the mask, was often accompanying the machine noise with her own vocal sounds that suggested that someone was quite unhappy.

One day, Roberta wandered into Yvette's room when the treatment was in progress, apparently seeing it for the first time. Roberta immediately thought that Carmen, who was always at Yvette's side during these treatments, was torturing Yvette. She evidently saw the mask as some diabolical device, and this notion was reinforced by what she must have thought were Yvette's cries or screams for help.

Roberta yelled at Carmen: "You wicked witch. Wicked witch. What are you doing to your mother?" Then she moved her entire body sharply and heavily against Carmen, attempting to shove her out of the way so that she could save Yvette. Carmen, though a much younger woman, found it necessary to call loudly for help. So powerful had Roberta become in her mission to relieve her friend, Yvette, from the torture of a Witch that it took two staff members to escort her out of the room.

This could be a lesson to those who believe that all dementia sufferers are withdrawn from the world, absorbed only in themselves, without the sensitivities that we possess. Sure, what Roberta apparently saw was unreal, but try to ignore that and focus instead on her passion to save a good friend, a "sister" of hers, Carmen's "mother", in this confined and hidden place of lost memories.

14

During the last few weeks of her life, Yvette loved to play a knee game with me. I was seated on her red sofa and she was in her chair, with her feet free of the foot rests, which had been swung back to the sides. Then Yvette, facing me, would move forward with foot movements until our knees touched. We would then inch even closer to each other, often with one of my knees sliding in between her knees several inches. We locked our legs together, hers-mine-hers-mine.

Why did we do this? Well, throughout our lives, we had often been physically close to each other. I had my arm around her or I walked with her arm in arm or we hugged or we held hands or we sat close to each other or . . . Now, in the last few years, Yvette was either in bed by herself or she was seated in her chair by herself. And I was by myself. Sure, we could still hold hands, and I could put my arm around her shoulders (though that wasn't easy), or pat her with my hand on her shoulder or arm. But it wasn't as intimate, it wasn't like a hug. So apparently we both felt good about interlocking our legs, and pressing them tight, one against the other. Then I usually rubbed the calf muscles of her legs, pretending to give her a massage on each muscle. She appeared to enjoy that. Carmen told me that, when we were thus engaged, staff members cautioned each other to stay away. Imagine that! I'm 94 and Yvette was 92, and we were both fully dressed. What's your problem, guys?

15

Yvette had to endure daily several breathing treatments she did not like, some of them during the night -- every night -- when she was sleeping. She was given medications several times a day and at night. At least three times daily she was lifted by two people from her bed onto her chair. Then as many times the other way. She was upset each and every time this took place. She was lifted onto the toilet chair and wheeled into the bathroom a few times daily. In the bathroom, while on the toilet, Yvette usually voice-cried, as two people were in there with her, while she was trying for a bowel movement. During the night, when she could not get up, her diaper had to be changed. It was changed again in the morning. Despite that, Yvette managed to be continent during the day. Could you have kept night practice separate from day practice as Yvette did? When she was ill, she had to have her vital signs recorded daily, blood pressure taken which she hated, temperature, pulse rate, oxygen level in her blood. There were X-rays. Her meals were fed to her every day, and during her final months she could have only puréed food. During these months, she often had to eat in her room, rather than at the dining table, where there was a lot more going on. Yet despite all of these daily inconveniences, annoyances, intrusions, and distasteful and frightening things, Yvette continued to smile at her aides, at Carmen, and at me on many occasions, almost daily. She laughed at jokes and at silly things to entice her to laugh. She wasn't, by any means, always happy, but she was in a good mood more times than she had a right to be. And almost to the very end, she enjoyed her food and beverages. Enough times to matter, she said "Thank you" to anyone who had done something for her. Besides dearly loving her, I also came to admire her greatly for the happy qualities she revealed under duress, under stress.

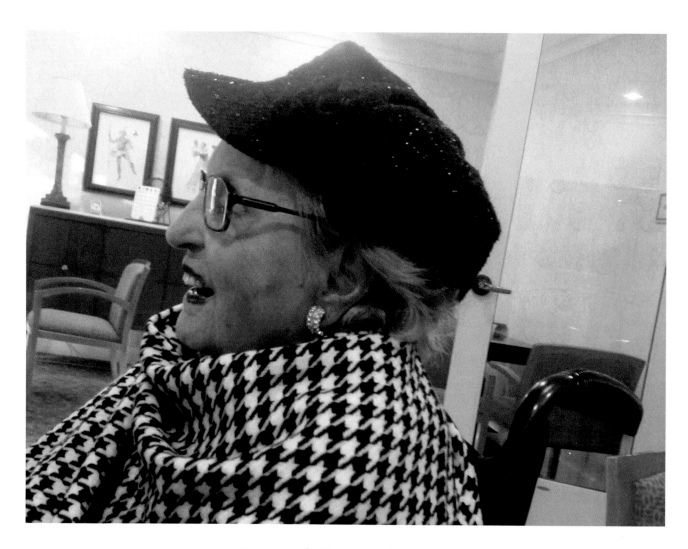

Yvette with New Shawl and Cap

16

Yvette had eaten her dinner in her room, Carmen as always feeding her. Yvette had eaten a very fine dinner, taken a short nap, and was now looking out her window at a small passing parade of bicyclists, a few pedestrians, some cars going in and out of the underground garage of Ronald McDonald House, a garbage truck, a Stanford bus, a dog or two. Yvette was seemingly making the best of these movements to and fro by paying attention to them all.

Then Yvette, for the first time since she was confined to her transport chair, crossed her legs, left over right, leaned back in a relaxed way, and grinned at Carmen with a look that seemed to say "You know, I haven't a care in the world." Carmen had never seen those crossed legs before. Or that accompanying carefree look. So she grabbed a camera and, with some difficulty establishing a good position, got a few shots of this beautiful woman, whose life was almost a continuous round of medications, treatments, X-rays, illnesses and recoveries, and dozens of other annoyances and irritations. She got a few shots of this courageous and happy resident of Memory Support, who had decided that right now she would throw her many cares away and enjoy to the full these precious moments.

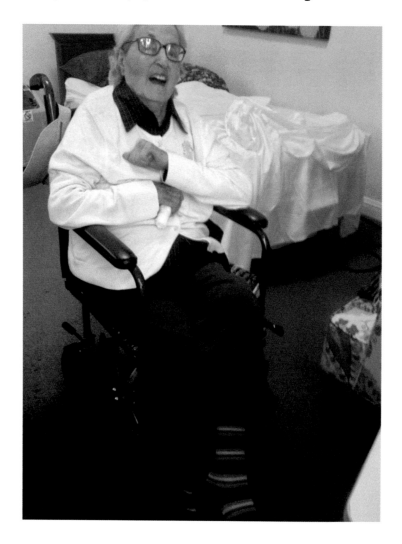

Crossing Her Legs

17

Yvette was with Carmen almost every day for over 2 1/2 years, and yet she never called Carmen by name. She certainly knew her name, for if someone, coming into the room, called out "Carmen," Yvette would turn her head toward where Carmen was located. Carmen many times jokingly told Yvette "I am Carmen." But Yvette did not bite. In fact, she never, while in Memory Support, said "Jack" to me directly, though she would ask Carmen about me, like "Where is Jack?", when I was walking behind them. But she never said "Hi Jack". And yet, with only two exceptions, my name was the only one she ever said. She would occasionally, when reading name tags, say the person's name. The second exception was really funny, as she began calling Carmen "Chicken." When Carmen first heard this she asked Yvette if she really thought her name was Chicken. Yvette's response was to laugh. And that's the way it continued: Yvette looking at Carmen and saying "Chicken," Carmen pretending to be greatly offended, and Yvette laughing. Carmen and I believe that my darling wife simply found a way to have fun.

18

Yvette slept with lots of pillows. Each pillow had a colorful pillowcase. There were red ones, purple beauties, yellow, green, and pink displays, and more. Two pillows were under her head. Two were on each side of her. When she was on her back, another was between her legs. Our Beauty Queen was decked out with seven colorful pillows, which we all knew were proper for a Queen. Five for a Princess, but seven for the Queen. Proper, too, for keeping her in new positions during the night, as we tried to prevent regal bed sores.

For a long time, our Queen accepted this pillow arrangement. But any Queen, when told what to do a hundred times each day -- when to eat, when to nap, when to get up or go to the bathroom, when to do this and that -- would naturally, in the end, rebel in order to show the motley crowd who was boss. There are any number of ways to rebel. Our Queen Yvette, finally fed up with all those damn pillows and all the other orders from her lowly subjects, found her own way.

All seven pillows in place, lights dimmed, time to go to sleep. Carmen has said goodnight to the Queen. Carmen leaves. Our Queen sends, with the sweep of an arm, one pillow flying toward the window. Another lands on the sofa. Two hit the armoire and fall on the floor. A fifth seems shot out of a cannon and is flattened against the far wall. Our Queen keeps the two under her head. Royalty requires a good night's sleep.

19

As I noted before with sadness, the Beast took away most of Yvette's ability to speak. Yet during this mostly-silent period, Yvette did say many things, though most of these remarks were inarticulate. Most of those that were understandable were in only a couple of words. Many times, Yvette said "Thank you" to someone who had just done something for her. She also could say "Nice" when she appreciated something. She spoke names a few times, like "Ernesto". She referred to me as Jack. "Let's go," was a favorite of hers for quite some time. She greeted strangers at the Shopping Center with "Hello." She told us, a few times, what signs said, like ATM or Macy's. She appeared to read many signs we passed on our walks, though silently. "All right" was another favorite of hers.

Occasionally, however, Yvette would come out with somewhat longer statements, and Carmen and I would rejoice. One day, when we were seated at a table in Co Co La, Yvette, looking at Carmen, said clearly: "Nice table. Nice place." She had been smiling, looking around, enjoying a cappuccino, observing the people coming and going, and those four words were meant to sum up her happiness at that moment. Because those happy words came after two or three days of agitated- restless behavior, they hit Carmen and me in a way that brought tears to our eyes. Yvette was happy, and she was able at that moment to tell us so. Couldn't have been a better day for us.

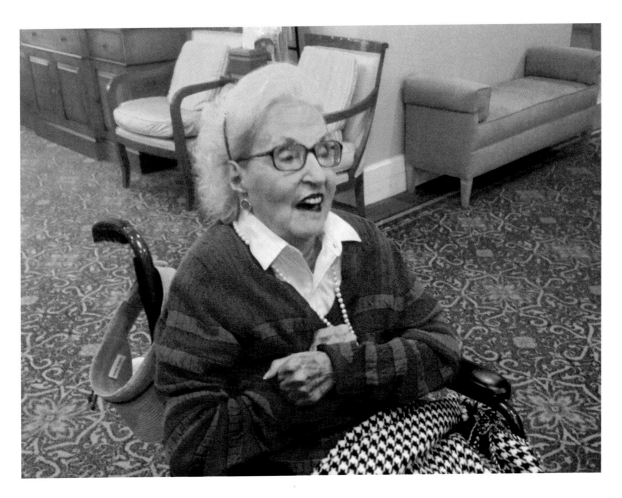

A Little Laugh

Every once in a while Carmen would mention me to Yvette in connection with something then going on. For instance, one afternoon when a friend had her laptop out, Carmen said to Yvette, "You know, Jack is an expert with computers." Yvette immediately replied: "I don't think so." Then she started to laugh. She couldn't have been more right. She used that phrase several times in the last five months, always almost singing it. "Think" was a few notes higher than the other words.

Not long ago, someone brought me a small glass of wine and a cookie in the Care Center's Grand Salon. When Yvette saw the cookie, she said: "Give me back my cookie." Now that went back several weeks, when I did take a cookie from her at the dining table in Memory Support 2. At that time, Yvette had made exactly the same remark. Here it was, several weeks later, but the cookie this time was not hers. Still, Yvette, dementia and all, remembered when the cookie was actually hers and what she had said, and so she applied it to the present situation. Not only was this a nice, clearly-said sentence, but it was also quite a memory for someone in Memory Support.

Carmen wheeled Yvette to the Stanford Shopping Center many times before and after her pneumonias. I was always along, usually walking behind with my small grocery cart. We would settle down at La Baguette. One morning, after I had taken my seat next to Yvette, she turned to me and, with a smile, said: "Thank you for coming along." On another day, I stayed at our table while Carmen wheeled Yvette around the Center. When they returned 20 minutes later, Yvette asked me: "Where have you been?" On still another occasion, Yvette, on seeing me seated next to her, said: "You look nice." One morning, on our way over to the Center, we were waiting with others at Sand Hill Road for the pedestrian crossing sign. When it came on, two other people stepped out in front of us, and Yvette shouted at them: "What about us?" There was the morning when, as we started out of the Care Center, we encountered another group. Yvette said to them: "This is my husband who is a professor."

Carmen and Ernesto often, in a corridor, helped Yvette stand up from her transport chair, and then, one on each side of Yvette, they would walk her down the corridor. One afternoon, Ernesto told Carmen that he was really too tired from his day's work to walk Yvette. When Yvette overheard that, she told Ernesto: "I'm going downhill." Evidently, she meant that his decision was a setback for her.

When Yvette was told that she had on a pretty sweater, she replied: "I have better ones."

All right, my friends, you are now sound asleep. When you wake up, you might like to know that every one of those "sayings" of Yvette, every single one of them, made our day.

20

Yvette could laugh and laugh and laugh. In three years, Carmen and I observed perhaps 35 residents in the Memory Support units and we never saw or heard anyone else laugh. Only Yvette. Each day we saw a few residents smiling now and then. But the norm was no or little facial expression. Yvette laughed easily -- at things we said that tempted her to laugh, at our own facial expressions, at the sheer joy of starting out to the Shopping Center, at small children chasing pigeons at the Center, at the pleasure of seeing friends, frequently at Carmen's remarks, and Ernesto could often make her smile, then laugh. Yvette usually laughed at André Rieu's marching band coming into the concert hall, as she viewed it on our iPads. She loved his Three Tenors, and laughed when she saw them. She laughed at some of my stories about my mother inviting her to a Thanksgiving dinner, about how we got married, and much else of our early married life. Carmen and I were sometimes surprised by a laugh from Yvette when we were talking to each other, not realizing that Yvette was listening. Yvette saved many of her laughs for Gigi, the granddaughter of Lindsay Morgenthaler.

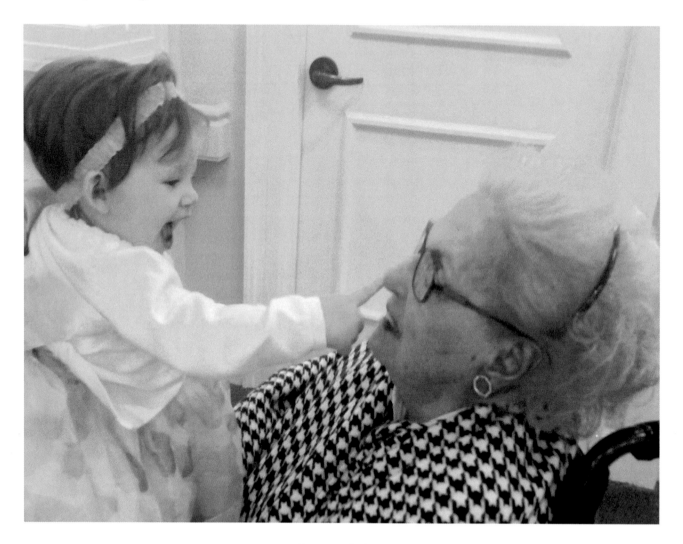

Gigi and Yvette

This is someone deep into dementia who somehow managed to retain, and was allowed to use occasionally, a sense of humor coupled to joy and a feeling of happiness. Yvette laughing and laughing -- Carmen, I, and many others will never forget her in those happy moods.

21

Yvette and I went to the San Francisco Symphony and Opera for about 40 years. Since I knew that sort of music was in her ears, Carmen and I often played classical music and operatic arias for Yvette on our iPads during lunches and dinners in her room, and in afternoons in the Card Room. We found that Opera duets, trios, quartets especially appealed to her. She also loved the Three Tenors -- Pavarotti, Domingo, and Carreras. The Chopin Nocturnes were also high up. But to our surprise her top choice during the last several weeks of her life seemed to be The Four Seasons by Vivaldi. (This, of course, was out of our narrow selection.) Each of these violin concertos evokes its season. We start with spring, go to summer, then autumn and winter. YouTube has several offerings of this composition, some video with orchestra and some audio with beautiful pictures. It lasts for about 42 minutes, which was just right for meal times. Carmen put it on softly, as background music, but had the iPad placed so Yvette could easily see the screen. This did not distract Yvette from the enjoyment of her food, which was always a given. But coupled to her eating pleasure was her delight for the music she evidently loved. Carmen or I would sometimes suggest that this must be, let's say, summer, because you can hear the summer thunderstorm. Or other such remarks. And Yvette appeared interested. It was this music that lit up Yvette's eyes, that drew her attention, like nothing else that we found could.

22

During her last four months, Yvette frequently had to have her oxygen level and pulse rate taken. There is a small instrument that records both. A thumb fits neatly into its tiny jaw, and it's the thumb that provides the two numbers that are shown on the face of this instrument -- let's say 97 and 85. The first number tells you about your lungs, how much oxygen they are getting into your blood. 85 tells you about your heart.

As I've noted a few times, Yvette's fingers and thumbs were curled into fists, so it was too difficult to fit this instrument around a thumb. Instead, Yvette's right big toe was used. Not the left one because she could kick up a storm with her left leg. Carmen got these numbers whether Yvette was seated in her chair or lying in bed.

Yvette never liked any of the tests for vital signs. Accordingly, we always tried to tell her stories or to calm her in other ways when they were going on. During the oxygen-pulse one, I told her what terrific circulation of numbers she had throughout her body that allowed us to get two numbers from her big toe. All her numbers, I told her, went round and round, so it was necessary for her to be patient until the numbers we wanted had circulated down into her foot and then into her big right toe.

Yvette listened and did calm down the first three or four times I did my gig. After that, she gave me the equivalent of a yawn and squirmed and kicked, sometimes sending the small instrument high into the air. You need lots of oxygen for that.

23

I previously told you that the Dementia Beast took away Yvette's ability to walk. That was gradual. Years ago, Yvette began falling from time to time. Then I found she would not -- could not -- go down escalators. Then she had trouble sitting down and getting up. Finally, while in Memory Support for less than a year, her legs wouldn't hold her up anymore. At that point, we got a transport chair for her, and for about two years she was confined to that.

Everyone, doctors and nurses and aides, told us that that was that. But you know what? If it had not been for those horrible pneumonias, we think we would have had Yvette walking again -- with a walker, to be sure, but walking again. We started our mission right away. Before getting Yvette out of bed each morning, Carmen rubbed her legs and then moved them, bicycle fashion, backwards and forwards. In her chair, we encouraged Yvette to move her chair forwards and backwards with her feet and legs. Yvette did this willingly throughout the day, month after month, on her own initiative. She was persistent, determined. Next, we bought bicycle pedals for her that sat on the floor in front of her chair, and allowed her to pedal, as though on a bicycle. This, too, she liked and used frequently. During this time, as well, Carmen and Ernesto, or Carmen and Melanie, on many days, stood Yvette up, and with them on each side of Yvette they all walked along the long corridors. Yvette was doing very well walking, with her aides, long distances. Carmen was elated that Yvette was "getting lighter", that is she was herself walking more heavily, making it lighter on them. She was not being dragged along. She was walking, and walking quite a ways -- and, what's more, she wanted to. She was determined to walk again.

Our next step was to get Yvette a sturdy walker and teach her how to walk with it, without any help from Carmen, Ernesto, or Melanie. We were looking for one, and then her pneumonias struck. Bango. We were back to "that is that." After her recoveries, we started in again-- slowly, slowly. But the Beast did not give us enough time, for he quickly found a way to kill our Darling. And, then, that really was that.

24

Yvette may have forgotten a lot, but she remembered well how to play games with us, and to enjoy doing so. One game Carmen and I called Ouch! Early on, one of us or both squeezed Yvette's hand too hard, causing her to say Ouch! We would quickly apologize and promise not to do it again; we promised to hold her hand more gently next time. I know that, despite these promises, I was guilty of squeezing too hard a few more times. More Ouches! More apologies.

Then Yvette began her game with me. I would reach for her hand and, before I had done no more than barely touch it, we would hear Ouch! And a little smile might creep into this fun. The game even moved to the absurd, for I heard the Ouch! when my hand was still inches from hers. Ouch! Then a little laugh from our prankster.

I marveled at how someone with serious dementia could, nevertheless, retain this sense of fun, and, moreover, seem to know by her little laughs that she may have gone too far. Deeper thoughts aside, we loved this game that my dear wife had dreamed up and enjoyed so much. We played Ouch! nearly to the very end. Fun!

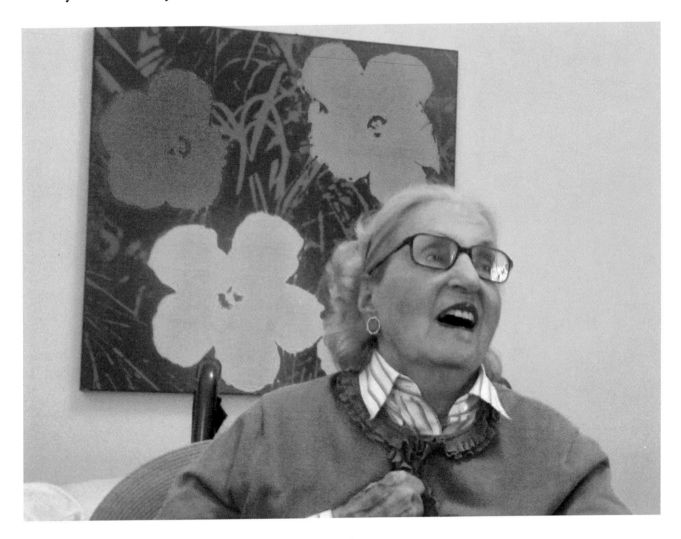

Prankster

25

In 1 1/2 years of trying, I never succeeded in getting Yvette to say yes or no to a simple question. I told her many times that, if she would answer yes or no, Carmen and I could help her greatly, make her life better, happier, and healthier. Yvette, do you have a headache? Do you want to go to the bathroom? Do you have a toothache? Would you like your nap now? Do you feel okay? An answer of yes or no seems simple. Yvette, just say yes or no, and that will help us to take care of you so much better. Yet, in 1 1/2 years, not once did Yvette respond to my plea.

As I've noted a few times already, the horrid Dementia Beast had taken away most of her ability to speak. Yvette must have had a very hard time in speaking even a single word. And yet, as I also described previously, from time to time she produced quite a few words, many, to our ears, quite wonderful. But, no yes or no to a simple question.

Was Yvette just being stubborn? Could she have answered but simply decided a few dozen times not to? I'm not sure. That's possible, for she didn't respond either to my request simply to shake her head yes or no. However, what I think is more likely is that Yvette found it very hard to answer any question on demand. She spoke only when all the conditions in her brain were right. Everything had to be lined up perfectly. Perhaps, also, there were certain words and phrases easier for her to say. This may have been so the several times she responded verbally to something taking place at that moment, like "Thank you." But usually she could not. She frequently knew what was going on around her. But seldom could she tell us any little bit of what she knew. Yvette probably wasn't being ornery. Instead, she might have been terribly frustrated by not being able to meet my simple demands. If that were so, I regret that I kept at it so much.

26

Yvette's attractive clothes were scattered among her friends, the workers in Memory Support, just as her ashes were scattered in the friendly waters by the Golden Gate. Those who loved her, and their sisters, daughters, and mothers, will, in my mind's eye, be Yvette herself as they display to the world her pretty and colorful hats, scarves, sweaters, shirts, blouses, pants, socks, and shoes, for years and years to come. We already have been shown such photos. Much better to her Memory-Support friends and their families than to all the strangers at Good Will.

27

Once or twice every week, the residents of Memory Support were entertained with sing-alongs. One of the songs the group sang frequently was You Are My Sunshine. This was always sung with joy in the air.

You are my sunshine, my only sunshine.
You make me happy when skies are grey.
You never know, dear, how much I love you.
Please don't take my sunshine away.

However, every time I heard that refrain, I had a feeling of foreboding. My sunshine was surely going to be taken away, and I would be left with nothing -- for she was my only sunshine. As I said, joy was in the air as the song was sung, but it made me so very sad.

Well, my sunshine, my Beauty Queen, my dear Yvette was taken away, just as I feared. I have attempted here to bring her back with my memories of her. I know that I cannot really bring back Yvette, but I hope I have succeeded in doing another good thing -- and that is telling you why she was loved so very much by me, by Carmen, and by many, many others. All of us miss her incredibly.

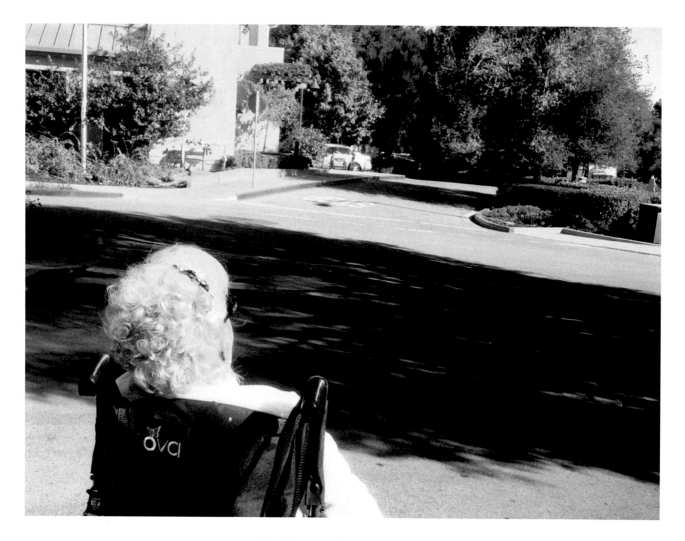

Looking and Going Away

28

Carmen Galindo was with Yvette for over 2 1/2 years. I was with Carmen, as she cared for Yvette, for several hours each day during that entire time. During the last 6 months of Yvette's life, Carmen cared for Yvette for 14 hours a day, every single one of those days.

Yvette died on December 9, 2014. That left Carmen and me alone. Goodbye Carmen? Goodbye Papa Jack? Of course not.

We had been through too many awful periods, too many happy times, just too much together, to part now.

We were alone and so we needed each other. We needed to tell each other many stories about Yvette, to relax together and try to recover the bodies and minds we once had, to plan how to tell the world about this courageous, beautiful, and admirable woman we loved so much.

We're together for therapy. We're together now because Yvette still lives in our hearts.

Printed in the United States
By Bookmasters